ORAL PRESEN
IN MEDIC

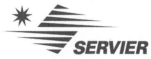

SERVIER

This publication has been made possible
through an educational grant from Servier

Springer

Paris
Berlin
Heidelberg
New York
Barcelona
Hong Kong
London
Milan
Singapore
Tokyo

A. Fingerhut, F. Lacaine

ORAL PRESENTATION IN MEDICINE

Abe Fingerhut, M.D., FACS, FRCS
Associate Professor of surgery at Louisiana State University
Centre Hospitalier Intercommunal
10, rue Champ-Gaillard
78303 Poissy Cedex, France

François Lacaine, M. D. PhD, FACS
Professor of surgery at Pierre et Marie Curie University (Paris VI)
Hôpital Tenon
Service de chirurgie digestive et générale
4, rue de la Chine
75970 Paris Cedex 20, France

ISBN 2-287-59686-0

Springer-Verlag France
a member of BertelsmannSpringer Science + Business Media GmbH
© Springer-Verlag France 2002
Printed in France

SPIN: 10753883

CONTENTS

"You may fool all the people some of the time; you can even fool some of the people all the time; but you can't fool all the people all the time"

ABRAHAM LINCOLN

"Do as I say, not as I do"

BURKHART S,
Br Med J 1983;287:893

"It is just as important to present your work in a polished form as it is to conduct your research carefully. Making a presentation is an integral part of any research project, and it can be a stimulating exercise."

POLLOCK A, EVANS M,
Principles and Practice of Research
Springer-Verlag, New York, 1991

INTRODUCTION

Scientific knowledge may be communicated in the written form or orally. Written communication (medical writing) usually takes the form of original or research papers, which appear in scientific journals. Oral communication in medicine is usually made during a meeting and is often called a free paper. Oral medical communication abides by certain rules. The objectives of this book are to examine and discuss these rules.

Oral medical communication involves taking the floor to speak, whether it be as a speaker, the person who gives the talk in front of an audience, or as part of the audience, who can then ask questions or make comments. The go-between is called the *moderator.*

Some forms of oral communication are more specific to meetings with a large audience: free papers, panel discussions or roundtables, posters, and videos. Others are more characteristic of smaller audiences: hospital staff meetings, or literature update sessions. Educational talks have a didactic goal and resemble a lecture, for instance, in a course, or are closer to a case report, when they are given during a small class get-together.

For the sake of comprehension and ease of description, we will first deal with the free paper and preparation of slides because these are the most widely used methods of oral communication. This is characteristic of most of the techniques used for medical communication and will serve as the basis for our presentation.

THE FREE PAPER

Delivering a talk as a free paper involves four different steps:
1. The conception of the communication;
2. Production of the visual aids, which will serve as the vector of the communication;
3. Presenting the paper in front of an audience;
4. Discussion with that audience.

By conception of a medical communication, we mean putting together the scientific arguments in order to give an oral presentation. The most widely used visual aid is slides. Nowadays, electronic presentations are gaining in popularity. Presenting and discussing are related to theatrical techniques.

Although artificial in time and space, this structure – conception, production, presentation, and discussion – enables us to describe two sequences: the orator is first a "composer," in that he has conceived the communication and the visual aid, before he becomes the "interpreter" during his presentation to the audience and during the discussion with the audience. In his role as interpreter, he takes on two tasks: first as a "communicator," during the presentation, and next, as a "scientist," during the following session of questions and answers, which make up the discussion.

The orator and four steps in free paper presentations:
The orator is first a composer, conceiving the communication and the **visual aid.** He then becomes the **interpreter** of the communication in front of the **public,** and then a **"scientist"** during the **discussion** with the public.

1
CONCEPTION

Conceiving a free paper presentation is similar to thinking up an original research presentation and obeys the same rules as those in medical writing. As in a manuscript for publication, a free paper presentation should be constructed with the five-point "IMRAD" structure. The acronym stands for: Introduction; Material and methods; Results; And Discussion. In verbal medical communication, the discussion is replaced by a conclusion, which should trigger the debate, ie, the discussion with the audience.

> The **structure** of a free paper: "IMRAD"
> Introduction;
> Material and methods;
> Results;
> And
> Discussion (replaced here by a conclusion)

The conception of a free paper presentation involves a progression of steps and abides by several rules:

1. The goals of the communication should be defined by asking the question: what is the main message? This message should not be drowned or "diluted."

2. The author should make a list of 3 to 5 strong points contained in this message, in order to help in developing or reinforcing it during the presentation. These strong points should also help in the conclusion.

3. The author has to ask him- or herself how to get the "main" message across to the audience. Once "conceived," the talk takes the form of a text which should be written out.

The text can be written *out in full* or else be replaced by a simple outline; any and all intermediate forms are possible. Whether you actually write the text or not, and the way you write it (in full or outline), and whether you learn the text by heart or not, differs according to the type of presentation you are making and according to the language in which you are to give your talk, as well as your own experience with speaking in public. An 8-minute talk can easily be written down completely, while this is unlikely for a lecture lasting one hour.

Aside from some exceptional situations, as suggested below, it is usually not recommended to read the text in front of the audience, except, perhaps, in the case of very early experiences with speaking in a foreign language.

2
VISUAL AIDS

Most often, the visual aid used for a free paper is slides. The role of slides is to increase and/or accelerate the understanding of the spoken message. It has been said that we retain 20% of what we hear and 30% of what we see. Combining a spoken message with a visual aid more than doubles the understanding and recall. Slides are an excellent visual aid, but often they are not used well and/or to their full capacities, essentially because of their poor conception and/or because they are used as a goal in themselves. They cannot be a substitute for the spoken word, and hence should show as little written text as possible.

Slides are usually easy to make, especially when using the powerful and user-friendly software available nowadays, among which one of the most popular and widely used is *PowerPoint™*. These programs allow one to decide on the layout and then make a reproduction in the form of a photograph of the actual slide (most often a 35-mm film), which can be inserted into the slide frame. During the presentation, the information on the slide is projected on a screen using a slide projector. It is also possible to project the slides either directly from one's own computer (usually a laptop) or else by providing the organizers of the congress with a disk or CD containing the (virtual) slides.

The actual production of the slides, including the film processing and framing, usually takes some time, and this has to be taken into consideration when planning your talk. There are also instant solutions, either using a camera (Polaroid™, for example), capable of creating transparent photographs directly from the software or using modern photography shops, which also have equipment that can develop such films within an hour for four 36-exposure films.

The equipment necessary to project the slides is widely available. However, increasingly often nowadays, the video projector is the modern alternative to slides. Widespread use of digital cameras will probably accelerate this development. One undeniable advantage of this system is that the user can create his or her own slide portfolio inside his or her laptop, and from this slide bank, create and compose (and recompose) the presentation, as desired, and whenever necessary, within a very limited period of time. A second advantage of this system is the possibility of updating the information on the slides, from one presentation to the next as a result of the comments made or questions raised during the discussion period or according to new information gleaned from the literature. This advantage may become a disadvantage when the updating is done at the last minute and is not checked before the presentation. A third advantage is the possibility of "activating" the slide contents. It is thus possible to reveal information progressively, in small doses, line by line. Caution, however, must be exercised not to overdo it, because you do not want this to "contaminate" the message. The orator literally then disappears behind the "slide show." For presentations showing a surgical technique or another procedure, a video clip can be inserted directly into the electronic presentation.

Irrespective of the type of presentation, the traditional "slide" with its plastic or metallic frame or "virtual slide" images on the computer, to be projected on to a screen via a videoprojector, may be composed of words, tables, or figures. The latter includes graphs, drawings, schemes or photographs, such as X-rays.

While there is no ideal slide, there are some simple rules that we think are essential.

◾ DESIGN OF SLIDES

Avoid slides that are "full" because they contain too much data, color, and shading, and too many lines, and, for virtual slides, too many activations. Frames around the slide should also be avoided.

Slides are rectangular in shape. The long axis should be projected in a horizontal fashion (wider rather than tall); this is also called the "landscape" presentation. Slides that are taller than they are wide, the "portrait" presentation, should be avoided for several reasons:

1. Most screens are wider than they are tall (landscape) and therefore

2. The lower (or upper) part of the (portrait) slide will not be on the screen and so will not be read. These problems are increased when the screen is too low and/or the room is too small to allow the screen to be moved back.

The margins on the vertical and horizontal axes should be well balanced and not too wide, which might mean that the image or message is lost in the middle of the screen, or not too narrow, which could mean that part of the image is off the screen.

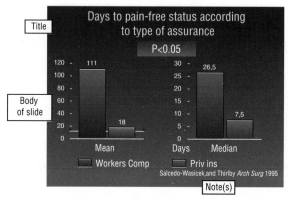

Fig. 1: A slide is made of a title, a body and notes.

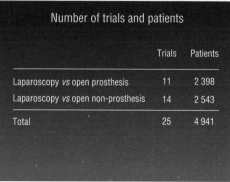

a

b

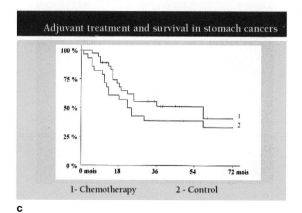

c

Fig. 2: Slides: a) text; b) table; and c) figure.

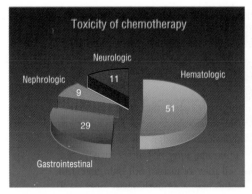

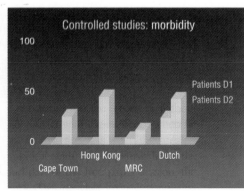

a

b

c

d

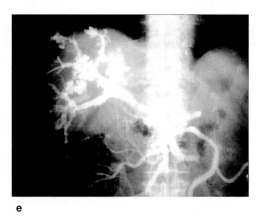

e

Fig. 3: Figure slides: a) pie chart; b) histogram; c) flow chart; d) drawing; and e) photograph (radiograph).

The rule should be to have *one idea* per slide. To abide by this rule, each slide should have a specific title, a main body, and, wherever necessary, one or two notes (Fig. 1).

As much as possible, slides should show objective data, such as tables, figures, or photographs, rather than text (words).

There are three types of slides: those that show *text, tables, or figures* (Fig. 2).

Figures can be graphs, diagrams, or photographs (Fig. 3). The most commonly used are X-rays, computed tomography (CT scans), sonography, magnetic resonance imaging, or pathology sections.

Slides showing text (words)

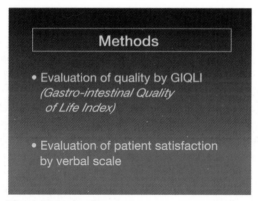

Fig. 4: Slide showing text.

As mentioned above, slides showing text (Fig. 4) should be avoided, but we will deal with them first. The reason for avoiding them is that text on a slide contaminates what is being said. The explanation is simple: the eye reads text much faster than the speaker can say it. Thus, the audience can assimilate and read text before they have the time to hear it. This contamination is even worse when the words uttered by the speaker do not correspond to what is written, thus leading to the recommendation that when text (words) is used, the speaker should stick to the text and avoid using synonyms or other words. This is especially important when the language used in not one's mother tongue because confusion can undoubtedly arise when the word on the screen is not heard.

Layout and characters used
Slides containing text (words) must adhere to specific rules.

Overall appearance

The general appearance of slides must be homogeneous. The color of the background, the font, or the color of the letters should not change from one slide to the next. The only exception to this rule is the use of bold type, italics, or underlining or changing the size or the color of some of text when the speaker wants to emphasize something. For instance, the degree of significance may be highlighted thus (**$P<0.0001$** or **$P\leq0.01$**).

Number of words and lines

We feel that it is artificial to set an absolute limit for the number of words per line or the number of lines per slide. Rather, these are determined by the duration of the projection of the slide. There is a need for a balance between the volume of information to be given and the duration of the presentation. The more lines there are, the longer the slide has to be shown. Occasionally, the organizers of the meeting themselves set these limits. Aside from this particular scenario (ie, imposed limits), we recommend that there be no more than six lines per slide. This excludes any notes such as references. When the information provided in the slides comes from the literature, the source of the information must be cited so that people in the audience can jot down the reference if they so wish. The best way to indicate this is to give the last name of the first author, without adding "*et al.*", the abbreviated name of the journal in italics, and the year of publication (eg, Smith, *Ann Surg* 1997). Generally, these references are placed in the lower right or left hand corner of the slide. The letters should be small, or at any rate much smaller than the size of the letters on the rest of the slide.

Enumerations

Enumerations must be justified on the left. They can be numbered or placed after bullets, a symbol that indicates the beginning of a line. Whichever you use, numbers or bullets indicate that the idea, argument, or general theme of what is written down has changed in relation to the preceding line. The use of numbers, however, implies a preference or order. If bullets are used, they should be small and inconspicuous, and one should avoid changing the style, color, or size from one slide to the next.

Font, size, case, and color of characters

We recommend the use of Arial or Times New Roman, because these are the fonts most widely used and most readily available on modern printers, and the letters are easily readable.

The characters should be sufficiently thick and tall. The size should be at least 24 points except for the references which can be as small as 14 or 18 points. Capital letters should be avoided. This is because lower case letters can be read more rapidly than capitals. Moreover, it is not necessary to start a sentence with capital letters except when the line is a whole sentence and grammatically correct. Furthermore, when needed in some languages, accents can be difficult to decipher when they are written in capital letters. Bold characters should be avoided, except to emphasize an idea or a sentence, as indicated above. In order to ensure legibility of the text, however, the font should be at least 24 points. Three-dimensional, shaded, and graduated characters should be avoided, whether for letters or numbers.

The best color for the characters -letters and numbers alike- is white or yellow, when the background is dark. Dark letters on a white background, often used in the past because they were the only ones available, should be avoided because the white background flashes and is tiring for the eyes. Red characters should be avoided, mainly because color-blind individuals cannot discern this color, and about 8% of people in an average audience are color-blind!

Interspace

For the best reading, the text should be compact and not spaced out. The spacing between lines is usually dictated by the font or characters that have been chosen. Beware of the temptation to modify the interspace, because increasing or reducing the character size can create smudging or will impinge on the adjacent line, making reading difficult or impossible. These errors in size are all the more deceptive because they are sometimes not apparent on the computer screen but appear on the final version of the slide!

Background

The color of the background should marry well with the characters (letters) and not obscure them. Gaudy or bright backgrounds such as red or yellow should be avoided. Blue and sometimes green are recommended. In practice, dark blue goes well with yellow and white letters.

Tables

The number of lines and columns in tables should also be limited for two reasons (Fig. 5). Too many lines and columns make the slide difficult to read and mean the speaker has to stay on the slide for too long, something which easily becomes boring for the audience. We recommend using a maximum of 5 to 6 columns and 6 to 7 lines. Lines around the table and especially framing the boxes should be used sparingly.

The heads of the columns and lines should easily be distinguishable from the data contained within the table. This may be accomplished by using different fonts, colors, and sizes, or using letters in italics or bold.

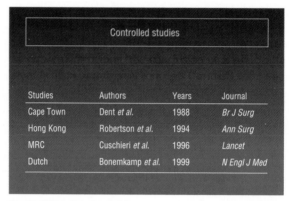

Fig. 5: Slide showing table.

Figures

Illustrations

Again, for reasons of legibility and the time needed to comment on illustrations (Fig. 6), the number of *lines*, the number of *parts* of pie charts, and the number of bars or blocks on histograms should remain within certain limits.

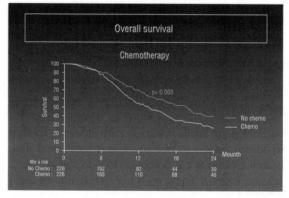

Fig. 6: Slide showing figure.

Line graphs

There should be no more than three to four lines on any one graph. The lines should be thick enough to be seen at a distance and the values, if shown, should be distinct from the actual lines. In addition, the confidence intervals for each point should be indicated. Legends should be provided for each axis.

Pie charts

There should be no more than five to six parts to each pie chart (Fig. 7). It is possible to separate the parts to make them more visible, and even to make them appear three-dimensional. If there are several small parts, it is best to group them together and label them as "others" or "miscellaneous."

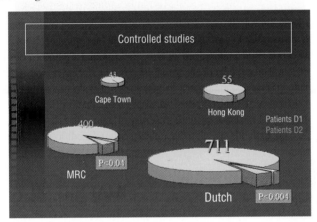

Fig. 7: Slide showing a pie chart.

Histograms

Vertical (columns) rather than horizontal (bars) should in line with the land-scape orientation of the slide (Fig. 8). Bars or blocks should be separated to make them more visible and, with most of the software available, it is easy to make them appear three-dimensional.

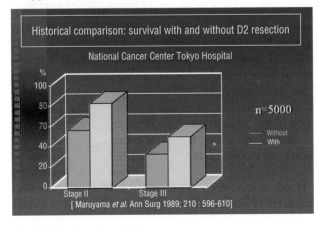

Fig. 8: Slide showing a histogram.

Flow charts

Flow charts (Fig. 9) are particularly suited to studies that relate to decision or treatment "arms." Each arm should provide details as to the composition of the different groups.

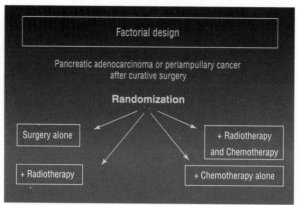

Fig. 9: Slide showing a flow chart.

Drawings

Remarks

When using three dimensions for pie charts and histograms, it is important to find the correct balance between the thickness of the lines and the spacing. This is relatively easy with the software available today as the bars or blocks or the parts of the pie charts can be rotated, or the three-dimensional effect can be decreased or increased in size. Once again, however, the more "optical effects" there are, the more the audience will be distracted from the message.

Drawings (Fig. 10) can help immensely in the understanding of a talk. They can be simple hand drawings or done by computer; they may be drawn from a data bank (or picture bank) or produced from suitable software.

Photographs

Photographs (Fig. 11), of which X-rays are one of the best examples, can be scanned and then inserted into the slide. There is also the possibility, if your computer is equipped with the necessary software, of downloading them directly from your source (eg, tape recorder, video recorder), or via the Internet.

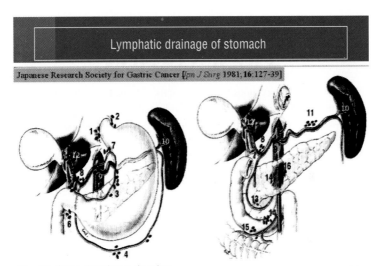

Fig. 10: Slide showing a drawing.

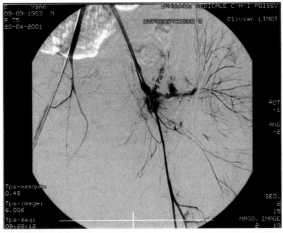

Fig. 11: Slide showing a photograph.

Legends

Legends can either be placed directly on (or near) the lines, the pie-chart parts, the histogram bars or blocks, drawings, and photographs or in a special box placed next to the actual chart. Ideally, the legends of the histograms should be horizontal. However, if there are many bars or blocks, the software may sometimes ignore one or two of the entries. In that case, you can tilt them slightly to get the entire legend on the slide. In this case, beware of tilting them too much, as the more they approach the vertical, the more difficult they become to read.

3
PRESENTATION

We have just seen the *composition* of the talk. The speaker was the "composer." The next step is *interpretation*, as the speaker now becomes an "interpreter." One should not forget that the audience will take notice of the speaker's qualities as an interpreter as much as his or her qualities as a composer. The communication takes center stage during the first role; the "scholar" or "scientist" stays in the background, until the discussion.

> The speaker changes his role.
> The "composer" becomes an "interpreter."

■ THE RULES OF PUBLIC SPEAKING

A free paper presentation usually lasts between 5 and 10 minutes, but most often, the talk lasts 7 to 8 minutes. The length of time left for questions and comments is usually 3 to 5 minutes, depending on the overall time allotted to each speaker. While the exact duration is usually dictated by the organizers of the meeting, this can nearly always be modified, sometimes by the organization itself, at other times by the chairman, according to local conditions or needs, for instance, a delay in the timing of a session would mean shortening the talk, or, on the contrary, the absence of one or more speakers would allow more time to be allocated. Once these limits have been determined and clearly announced by the chairman, strict adherence to the time limits is the primary concern of the speaker. The message must be as precise as the time in which to do it is short. Going over this limit is not acceptable to the organizers, the other speakers, or even to the audience. Speaking too long can create an unpleasant atmosphere in the room or on the stage (with respect to the chairman) and then be prejudicial to the message. Moreover, the longer the talk, the greater the risk that it will be interrupted before the conclusion, which is one of the strong points of the talk. The talk risks being incomplete and may end up being poorly understood or not understood at all.

■ SPEAKING

The speaker should speak as a communicator, in the same way that President Reagan was regarded when he appeared in public: as a great communicator, independently of the message that he wanted to get over. This role of being the communicator means that the speaker must forget that he is a medical doctor, which might seem a bit paradoxical. However, one must not forget that the most important accomplishment is to get the message over to the audience. In medical communication, there is a distinction to be made between getting the message across and the message itself. This means that when the speaker actually takes the floor he or she is more of an actor, rather than a doctor or specialist. A good communicator can be recognized by the way he or she can get a message across. A well-communicated message can be judged by the way the audience reacts during the discussion period. In fact, the discussion does not directly measure the *quality of the message*, which, of course, is very important, but *the quality of the way the message was transmitted*. Every one knows how political speakers, although we do not always agree with their message, can make such a convincing argument that we almost end up believing them.

Aside from these two elements related to the speaker (the quality of the presentation and the quality of the message), the interest stimulated in the discussion depends on the attitude of two other protagonists, the moderator and the audience (Fig. 12).

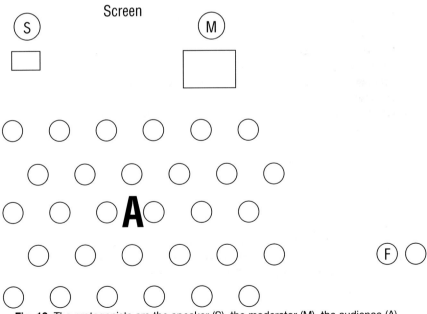

Fig. 12: The protagonists are the speaker (S), the moderator (M), the audience (A), and those who take the floor (F).

The speaker in relation to the environment

The stage is set. The speaker (S), the principal actor, enters the scene goes and to stand behind the lectern, usually placed at one end of the stage. On stage also is the moderator (M), behind, the screen, and in front, the audience (A).

The lectern and the instruments available to the speaker

The **lectern** marks the spot from which the speaker delivers the talk. Here there will be:

1. A small light source so that notes may be read, if desired.
2. The buttons necessary to run the slides (or the computer-assisted program).
3. A microphone. It is usually not possible for the speaker to stray much from the lectern and the microphone unless he or she has a neck, lapel, or wireless microphone and does not need to press the buttons personally to change the slides: in this case, the speaker can just say "next slide, please" to the projectionist, or sometimes this can be done with a wireless device. Some of the wireless handheld devices include a pointer. It is best to familiarize oneself with the different and various buttons in order to make sure that the talk goes as smoothly as possible.

The position of the speaker is somewhat "triangular," at an angle to the *moderator* and the *audience*. The speaker should directly address the *moderator* at the beginning and the end of the talk; at all other times, he or she faces the *audience*.

The screen is usually at the back of the stage, at the front of the room or auditorium, at some distance from the podium or lectern. It is very important for the speaker to become familiar with the layout of the room or auditorium, by visiting it, whenever possible, well in advance before the talk is scheduled. The *pointer* is the intermediary between the speaker and the screen. It may be either a light or a laser.

The special role of the pointer

The ideal situation is when the speaker can stand on the podium, behind the lectern, easily and comfortably speak into the microphone and from there see the screen, while at the same time being able to look at the audience without turning his or her back on them.

Problems arise when the place for the speaker is small and he or she is forced to move around on the stage to see or to show something on the screen. In this case, the speaker is obliged to find some solution to be able to negotiate between the lectern, the controls on it, and the screen while still making the audience his or her priority. The all-important link here is the pointer.

Correct use of the pointer includes the following:

1. The pointer should never be used continuously. This would quickly degenerate into what is called the "mad-moth syndrome," where the light darts all over the screen and back and forth or hovers on the word that is under scrutiny, or else remains on some irrelevant part of the screen, or worse on somebody else.

2. The pointer must be used judiciously, making sure that there is a relationship between what is being shown (pointed at) and what is being said at that time.

3. This means that the speaker has to choose the most appropriate spot on the podium, from which the screen can be seen correctly, and still stay in visual and audible contact with the audience. It may not always be possible to meet these ideal conditions, for example, in the case of a microphone that is too far away and/or cannot be moved around the podium.

> *To emphasize the key elements and enhance the understanding of the message, the speaker uses the light pointer or laser, instead of a stick.*
> The pointer is the physical link between the speaker, the audience, and the screen.

The pointer is a valuable tool for the speaker, because he or she uses it to show the elements he or she wants to emphasize, or is talking about. However, while using it the speaker should not ignore the audience. Priority must be given to the audience, and in particular, the speaker's voice must always remain audible. It may become necessary, because of the setup on the podium, to ask the technical staff (or the moderator) to turn the volume up or turn the microphone toward the speaker. The speaker should never lose visual or audible contact with the audience.

The beginning of the presentation: starting to speak

The action begins as soon as the moderator calls the speaker to the podium. The speaker has to make his or her entry, and then address the audience to gain their attention. One way of limiting stage-fright is to fix ones' eyes on the podium, make one's way up to the lectern and think of nothing in particular, while appearing *determined*. In addition to getting rid of any emotion and calming down, concentrating on the podium will allow the speaker to avoid any unnecessary footwork or tripping. One thing to remember is that sometimes the speaker has to approach the podium in the dark. This is another reason why the speaker should be familiar with the layout of the room and in particular with the podium and the best way to get there beforehand.

Next, the speaker stands behind the lectern breathes deeply, looks intently at the audience and then at the moderator. With this glance, the speaker assesses the situation, becomes aware of his or her overall task calmly, and therefore gains the confidence necessary to go on. This phase of the talk is a pause, a time of silence, which should last a few seconds. The speaker has to take advantage of this time to place the different instruments (pointer, controls) within reach. It might also be the moment when someone from the technical staff pins the lapel mike onto the speaker and/or sets up the computer. During this pause, the audience takes advantage of the "break" to get ready for the new talk.

As soon as the speaker has finished his or her preparations, the talk begins. Right from the very first word, the speaker's voice should be steady, loud, and audible. Each sentence has to be punctuated with quiet breathing, neither too short nor too long, clearly separating each sentence from previous one. This short pause can be used, provided the audience is sufficiently visible, to measure the impact the speaker is having on the audience. Capturing the audience is not a question of self-satisfaction. Visual contact with the audience is necessary to assess their reaction and can be used to modify tactics as required, at any time during the talk. In general, the speaker must be conscious of the fact that the audience is not hostile. Even if the speaker's voice is shaky or uncertain at the beginning, this does not mean that the speaker will be poorly judged by the audience, especially since voice problems should improve as the talk goes on, provided the speaker follows the simple recommendations found in this book. As indicated above, the speaker should be familiar and well versed with the talk: reading notes, or worse, the entire text, is not recommended. In the setting of a free presentation, notes are difficult to consult and continual consultation of them will lead, at one point or another, to some degree of dependency which the speaker will have difficulty in overcoming. The audience will be able to pick this up quickly. If the bulk of the talk is well known, this makes things easier, because the speaker can then concentrate exclusively on the way the talk is to be given.

The two ends of the presentation: the introduction and the conclusion

The introduction and the conclusion are two key moments: what is most important here is the contact between the speaker and the audience.

This is why we think that the introduction, and also frequently the conclusion, should be delivered with the lights on, without visual aids. We personally think that visual aids (slides or computer images) are a hindrance rather than a help at this particular time of the talk.

Introduction

After the moderator has announced the title of the communication, the speaker presents himself or herself to the audience, speaking without slides, with the lights on, and affirms his role of a *communicator*, delivering a scientific message to the audience. A short introduction is not only desirable for the clarity of the presentation, but constitutes a key moment in the presentation when the speaker can "set the scene" relating to the background of the topic of his or her talk. All too often, the audience is plunged directly into the dark, with the first, stereotyped phrase "Can I have the first slide, please?" often before the speaker has taken a look at the audience. This bad habit is so common that often the projectionist switches off the lights and shows the first slide even before being asked to do so!

Conclusion

Chronologically, of course, the conclusion takes place at the end of the communication. It must be simple and concise, in order to stimulate a reaction in the audience, which can be measured by the intensity of the questions and comments.

The conclusion can basically be delivered in two different ways, but there is no general agreement as to how this should be done:

1. Some speakers prefer to ask for the lights at this moment and finish their talk without any visual aids, affirming the message with force and impact orally.

2. Others think that the essential points of the communication, as seen on a slide, will help the audience to remember the message. In this respect, these speakers usually read the conclusion word by word. If there are several parts to the conclusion, they can be numbered according to their order of increasing or decreasing importance.

Development of the presentation: achieving a steady rhythm

Most often, the presentation is heavily dependent on visual aids. Harmony between the oral presentation and the visual aids is of the utmost importance.

Projection of slides

The number

How many slides? The absolute rule of "one per minute" appears to us, like many other restrictive rules, too strict because: 1) the time necessary to grasp the content of a slide is not the same according to whether it is an X-ray, a written message, or a table; and 2) as we have just seen, the introduction and sometimes the conclusion should be delivered with the lights on in the auditorium, without any visual aid.

The rhythm

It is important to determine beforehand how the slides work: is it by the speaker who presses a button on the podium or are the slides advanced by the projectionist, who should be prompted to do so, by the classic phrase "next slide, please," often just, "next"?

One slide every 20 to 60 seconds seems a good rate to aim for. Each change from one slide to the next should correspond to a moment of silence, especially when it is the speaker who does the changing from the podium. If not, announcing "next slide, please" to the projectionist fulfills the same role, providing a pause in the presentation. This key moment is particularly important at the very first slide; a similar pause should punctuate the last slide as well.

Time spent on the slide

It is up to the speaker to determine how long each slide is displayed, and the time he or she dwells on each part of the visual aid on the screen. It is also up to the speaker to determine the rhythm of the talk, and not the reverse, as with a video, whose timing has been set in advance. The time a slide remains projected on the screen depends not only on the amount of information it contains, but also on the duration of the comments that the speaker makes in support of the message. It is always possible, if necessary or desired, to go back to a previous slide, but beware of communication problems with the projectionist.

> Mention everything that is written on a slide, otherwise someone will want to know why something has been left out.

Title slide

Is there a place for the first slide with the title of the communication, the name of the authors and where they come from?

In our opinion, not shared by all, this type of first slide is a waste of time and pointless. Indeed, the information shown (the title of the communication, the name of the authors and their address) is:

1. Already found in the program.
2. Usually announced orally by the moderator, whose role is to present the communication to the audience.
3. Very often little understood because the speaker very rarely comments on the slide, "next slide, please" following hard on the heels of "first slide, please" with barely a pause for breath. Consequently, as the first slide goes by, time is actually lost for the presentation, which, as we have already said, should always follow a very tight time schedule.

If the author really wants to be recognized and/or show the names of the people who may have worked with him on the paper and thus thank them publicly, we would like to suggest that they do so on one of the last slides, shown either just before or just after the conclusion. If shown after the conclusion, this slide does not have be read; it can remain on the screen, while one waits for the discussion to start. In any case, as the speaker usually thanks the audience for their attention at the end of his talk, this marks the end of the message, a moment of transition, and the audience can read the names during the applause. In this manner, while the audience reflects on the message they have just heard, they can now associate the message with the names of the authors.

Another reason for not producing a title slide is, as we mentioned in the preceding chapter, that we believe that the introduction of a talk should be given with the lights on. The projection of a slide where the only information is the title, rarely if ever commented on, is actually an interruption in the scientific flow of the communication.

Double projection

A double projection is often seen as "something more." According to Barbier and Coiteux, visual communication is a monoconceptual phenomenon: "one image, one message." Double projection thus goes against this principle. The effect of a double projection is often pernicious, as the audience has to assimilate two images instead of one, often during the same period of time normally used for a simple projection. The audience loses time because they do not know which slide to read first, and their attention shifts from one slide to the other, especially when the speaker fumbles verbally while finding which slide he or she wants to begin with. Double projections can often result in repetition. Two slides, side by side, can be misleading: one slide can conceal part of the message of the other.

A double projection can be used to good effect in three settings:
1. The plan of the presentation can be put on one side, remaining there throughout the presentation, as the speaker scrolls through the actual presentation on the other.
2. In a foreign country, in which the audience does not speak the same language as the one in which the presentation is being made, one slide can be the translation of the other.
3. Illustrations (drawings, figures, and graphics) are projected on one screen while the corresponding text appears on the other.

If, in spite of our reticence, a double projection is still being considered, we recommend the following:

1. Make sure in advance that the room is equipped for a double projection (two slide projectors, two screens, enough space in the room or the auditorium so that everyone can easily see both screens).

2. Determine the order of projection of each slide set with numbers on one side and corresponding letters on the other (for example: 1 and A, 2 and B, 3 and C, etc), in order to be able to place the slides in the correct order (and also if someone mixes them up at the last moment).

3. Inform the moderator and the projectionist that you are going to use a double projection.

4. Find out in advance how the slides work: whether there are one or two buttons, which button corresponds to which screen (side), etc.

Animation

Animation is the term given to the effects that computers now allow to be added to the slide show. PowerPoint™ software is particularly useful and will serve as an example. Use of animation can add much to the presentation, a judicious intermediate between the classic slide show and the video. When used inappropriately, however, animation can lead to disasters that must be avoided.

Transition

The change from one slide to the next is called the transition, ie, how the slide appears on the screen or disappears from it. Slides may appear or disappear vertically or horizontally, starting in the middle, from the top, bottom, right or left.

Special effects

By special effects we mean the way the information on the slide appears on the screen. Once again, there are several possibilities. The lines can be made to appear one line after another, to appear with a sweeping motion or with a "checkerboard effect," etc. During the projection, these different effects can be activated by using the "enter" key or the "down" or "right" arrows.

The animation can be personalized as well with a myriad of combinations. This is done using the Powerpoint™ software by opening the "slide show" window and then choosing from the drop-down menu the "custom animation" command. With this window, you also can find the "after animation" effects, which allow certain words or boxes to be erased once they have appeared and been read.

In practice

Whatever the type of animation chosen, the effects have to be programmed in advance. The relatively simple transitions and effects can be done either with the "slide sorter view" mode, or combined with the more complicated effects, by using the "slide show" window and "custom animation" commands. Once they have been programmed, the effects have to be triggered either manually, ie, the transition or effect will be produced when the above keys are pressed. The other way to do this is to program the changes automatically with the appropriate commands located in the "slide show" window. The effect takes place after one, two or several seconds, accordingly. The duration of exposure (with the transition) is also programmable. Also, a pointer, either an arrow or a pen, can be inserted and then used in the same way as the standard handheld pointer, being moved about the screen with the mouse. Other animated or automated possibilities such as video clips, recordings, and musical effects are also available. Apart from the video clips, however, these should be avoided.

Dealing with the information on the slide

While it is not always necessary to read everything word by word, all the key elements on the slide must be mentioned, in order for the message to be best understood. Generally speaking, all the information on the slide must be commented on, or the speaker should at the very least explain why this is not the case.

How to deal with errors on slides

What should the speaker do when an error crops up on a slide and it is too late to correct it?

Two different approaches are possible according to whether the information is wrong or there is a spelling error, and whether the error can lead to a misinterpretation of the information or not.

In the case of an information error, or one that could mislead the reader, the error should be pinpointed and commented on, and the correct information must be given. Excuses are not necessary. The error should simply be corrected by saying, for instance, this number should be "x" and not "y."

In the case of a typographical error, it is not always useful because of the loss of time to make any fuss about it. One can stress the correct word by raising one's voice when the incorrect word is reached, or by circling the word with the pointer.

Transition between the conclusion and the discussion

The conclusion has a dual role:

1. At the end of the presentation, the conclusion should summarize and condense the message(s).

2. The conclusion should also be a transition step between the information revealed in the presentation and the discussion that follows. The situation and the roles have changed. Under the direction of the moderator, the

speaker is no longer the only one to talk, but now also listens to the audience. The speaker who was the transmitter now becomes the receiver. However, the speaker should answer the question that has been asked, and avoid all digression or added information. In other words, the speaker should not take advantage of this part of the presentation to keep on talking.

Whether the talk ends by reading the conclusion on the screen or without any visual aid, the speaker enters into visual contact with the audience when he or she asks for the lights to be switched on. In any case, it is when the speaker says "Thank you for your attention" combined with the applause from the audience, that the transition with the second part of the free paper session, the discussion with the audience, takes place. The speaker may instead say: "Mr Chairman, I have now finished. I am ready to answer any questions you or the audience might have."

In reality, the transition between the presentation and the discussion is important. As we stated at the beginning of this book, the speaker's part in the free paper session is incomplete in itself (the "D" is missing from the classic "IMRAD" sequence). The discussion is in fact a logical and necessary follow-on to the presentation. Beginners always hope that there will be no or few questions, because they fear that the questions might be difficult to answer or embarrassing. This fear is often unfounded. Do not forget that a good presentation is one which solicits many questions and/or comments. How the audience reacts to your presentation depends on the originality of the presentation or on the advances it affords and much more rarely on their criticism of it.

> The dual role of the conclusion:
> • Summarizes the essence of the message
> • Transition between the presentation and the discussion

The end of the presentation

Ideally, the moderator and the speaker have met and talked before the presentation: the moderator has informed the speaker of the constraints and time limits of the presentation and the discussion period, as well as the last-minute modifications that may have occurred (one or several presentations may have been cancelled, the order has been changed, or sometimes a new presentation may even have been added). Notwithstanding, the speaker has to remain within the time limit that has been set. The moderator can, and should, stop the speaker from running over time. This situation should, however, be avoided because it is disagreeable for everyone: for the moderator because his or her role is to facilitate the proceedings for everyone, speakers and audience alike; for the speaker because the talk might be cut off or ruined at one of its most crucial moments, ie, the conclusion; and for the audience, as well, who do not know what to think: as the message is missing and there appears to be a battle as to who can get the last word in, they may be disappointed not to be informed about what they came for.

4
DISCUSSION

The speaker changes roles:
The **communicator** reverts to being the scientist

At the end of most types of presentations, the moderator informs the members in the audience that the talk is now open to questions or comments. Questions imply that there should be an answer, whereas comments normally do not. The duration and the number of these questions or comments depend on the time allocated to this part of the presentation, as well as the overall time remaining in the session.

The audience, by and large, is not hostile. However, this "entropy" should not stop people from saying what they think. This leads us to distinguish between two types of interventions when taking the floor (comments or questions): positive and negative interventions. Positive comments or questions are in agreement with the speaker. Thus, for example: "I have observed the same results, though with fewer patients, but I fully agree with Mr X..." Negative comments or questions should not be unfounded, but on the contrary, they should be well constructed. Thus for example: "You have shown by this retrospective study that treatment A is better than treatment B, but in the literature, there are at least two controlled trials that go against your conclusions. How do you explain this difference?"

■ THE ROLE OF THE MODERATOR

Good moderators are those who prepare in advance and play their role, irrespective of their experience in this kind of enterprise. They should be informed of the contents of each presentation beforehand, and one of the obligations of the organizing committee is to see that the moderator gets a copy of the abstracts in advance. Moderators, often chosen because of their expertise on the general topic, or for political or local reasons, should be informed of the latest developments and studies on the topic.

The moderator must make people (speaker and audience alike) abide by the rules. It is through his or her intermediary that the speaker comes before the audience, and once again, it is via the moderator that the audience comes into contact with the speaker.

The moderator is also a Master of Ceremonies and has the role of the leader. As stated above, the moderator has to make sure that everyone stays on schedule. When announcing the talk (and the person who gives it), he or she should also remind everyone of the time allotted for the presentation and the question time after. During the talk, the moderator has to make sure that every-thing goes as planned, and thus is responsible for starting and ending the discussion (questions and comments) within the allotted time.

It is essential that the moderator be present in the room before the time announced for the session, in order that, ideally, all the speakers involved can present themselves and indicate that they are present, what language they are to speak in, whether they are to give a single or double projection, and whether there is a last-minute change in who is giving the talk. This is especially important, when, for some reason or another, the name on the program does not correspond to the person who actually delivers the talk.

The moderator has the responsibility of opening the session. Apart from being a timekeeper, the moderator announces the title and duration planned for the talk and the discussion. The exact title and the affiliations of the authors should be clearly stated, as well the name of the person who is delivering the talk. During the talk, he or she must make sure that silence is maintained throughout the session. If there is a timer available, either with an audible or visible signal to the speaker, the moderator is responsible for making sure that the system is triggered. If not, the moderator must interrupt the speakers to remind them that their time is up. When the talk is over, the moderator thanks the speaker and invites the audience to ask questions and/or comment on the talk. If the audience does not react quickly, the moderator should be ready to intervene, either to ask a question or to make a comment. This will often suffice to trigger questions and comments from the floor. On the other hand, the moderator should not take advantage of his or her position to monopolize the questions or comments: priority must always be given to the audience.

As the timekeeper, and when the session gets behind schedule, the moderator must adjust to the situation much, making sure that the upcoming talks are not jeopardized or penalized; one way of dealing with a speaker who goes over the time limit is to say that as a result of this, there will be no time for questions and/or comments. By the tone of the moderator, the speaker should not do that again!

■ THE RELATIONSHIP BETWEEN THE SPEAKER AND SOMEONE ASKING A QUESTION OR MAKING A COMMENT

There are two ways of asking questions or making a comment to the speaker. Most often, once the moderator has opened the discussion part of the session, the person who wants to intervene either raises his or her hand, or stands in line behind a microphone placed in the aisle of the auditorium for that purpose. The person should wait politely until the moderator gives him or her the floor. In other situations, the potential questions and/or comments are written on a piece of paper, usually distributed with the program, and handed in to the ushers. The moderator then summarizes the questions and does the actual questioning himself. The question should be sufficiently clear because usually there is no possibility of direct intervention, and if the question is not sufficiently clear to the moderator it might not even be put to the floor.

Whether it is the moderator or a member of the audience who intervenes, the number of questions and/or comments for the speaker should be announced clearly. In general, comments should be made first and questions last. Due to time constraints, the number and, especially, the duration of the questions and/or particularly the comments should be kept as brief as possible. As an example, the intervention could be something like "I have two comments and one question ..."

The speaker should always be ready to jot down the comments and questions in order not to forget anything when replying. With this in mind, the speaker should remember to bring a piece of paper and a pen to the podium. These may be on available on the podium at the beginning of the session, but might no longer be there later on in the session.

Finally, if some aspect of the topic that the speaker is less familiar with is raised, but somebody else (a colleague or superior) whom the speaker knows is in the room has the necessary expertise to answer, this person can be called upon to respond. If this is the case, however, it is up to the speaker to introduce that person and explain why the person and not the speaker is answering. In general, this can be left to the end of the discussion period. As this exception to the rule changes the overall tone of the question and answer period, it may prompt the moderator to close the discussion.

How to ask questions

The question can be on the form of the presentation, for instance, some question about the methodology, or on the contents, for instance, the value or the consequences of the work. It might also be the moment to ask the speaker why he did not talk about or mention one or more details that seem to be important: "You say that there is no difference between treatments A and B, but you did not mention the statistical test you used."

This is a key moment during which the intervening person can shine and be noticed. Whatever the type of question, however, the goal is not to humiliate the speaker or put him in a difficult situation: the audience will always be aware of this. This is another reason why the speaker should not be afraid of the questions and the discussion period.

How to make a comment

Often some aspect of the topic may not have been dealt with by the speaker because of lack of time, not because of ignorance. The temptation to redress this omission from the floor might be overwhelming. The moderator must be aware of this temptation at all times and limit this accordingly. Indeed, the goal of the discussion is to qualify, or put into perspective the speaker's message, or, on the other hand, to put forward a counterargument, but not to make another presentation. This is something all members of the audience should keep in mind. If they think the omitted topic is that important, they should have thought of it before and made their own contribution as a free paper, and not take advantage of the discussion period during the scientific part of the meeting to do so! The moderator has a strong role to play at this moment by suggesting, politely but firmly, that the two individuals concerned (the person in the audience and the speaker) get together after the session to discuss the issue.

Comments do not usually require an answer. If the comments are in agreement with the conclusions of the presentation, this is a sign that the message has been transmitted successfully. A simple "thank you" is enough to acknowledge this. If, on the other hand, the comment is in disagreement with the conclusions, or appears to be an attack, it should be considered as a question, but never as a provocation. Each point of the comment can be answered, one by one, but very briefly. Everything should remain polite, short, and to the point. If the speaker has nothing to add, the moderator should take the cue and move on quickly to the next question(s) or comment(s).

THE LECTURE

The idea behind a lecture is to invite an expert to talk on a topic he or she knows particularly well. The choice of the topic is generally very much dependent on the person and their personality. Most often, the topic is one of the expert's hobby-horses. The more the topic is in the news, the higher the chances of being asked to make a presentation. It is up to the host to determine the topic, and to explain why he or she chose this particular person to give this particular talk. The reasons why someone is chosen may be because of a recent publication on the topic, or another presentation that the same person delivered previously, which seemed to have struck a chord with one or more members of the organizing committee, who happened to hear about the talk or even be in the audience. While the overall topic has often been set in advance and cannot be changed, usually the exact title is generally relatively free. The organizers should indicate to the speaker the type of audience that should be expected, because the nature of the talk depends on this.

Submitting a paper to a free paper session in a scientific meeting is a voluntary undertaking. What the speaker says and does in a free paper session is his or her own responsibility. When invited to give a lecture, the speak-er has a more passive role. Generally speaking, the person who delivers a talk is supported financially and entertained by the organizing party.

1
CONCEPTION

A lecture usually lasts for at least 20 minutes. The structure differs from that of the free paper in many respects. Compared with an original report, the organization of a lecture is simpler and is usually of the type: thesis, antithesis, synthesis. It should have an *introduction*, a *body (evidence)* and then a *conclusion*. As in a free communication, the goal is not to show off one's own knowledge, but rather to provide the audience with a message.

It is important to take the time for definitions at the beginning of the talk, according to the audience you are dealing with. Furthermore, the goals of the talk have to be set out clearly. One should say what the talk is about, but also what it is *not* about. Because of the structure and the balance that has to be achieved during the talk, it is important to calculate the time necessary to put forward and develop each idea.

Unlike a free paper presentation, the text does not have to be written out in full, if only because of its length. The presentation should be constructed according to a list of key words or phrases that the speaker has memorized. For this, brief succinct notes with these key words may be used. An elegant way to do this is, of course, to use some sort of visual aid, preference being given to an image rather than to words as a prompt.

Generally speaking, because the person who delivers a talk is an expert, it is usually unnecessary to rehearse beforehand. However, when the speaker is delivering a talk for the first time or when the speaker is uncomfortable for whatever reason (for instance, when the talk is in a language which is not the speaker's mother tongue), rehearsals are always a good idea. Two very effective ways of doing this are either to make an audiovisual recording of one of the rehearsals and/or, whenever possible, to rehearse in front of one or two friends or colleagues. Rehearsing as such will allow the individual giving the talk to feel comfortable and to be able to talk without hesitation, mistakes, or hindrance.

In any case, the speaker should avoid reading the entire talk. Its very length would make this an extremely monotonous experience (for everyone, including the speaker, the organizers and, of course, the audience).

> "When a speaker takes the floor holding sheets of paper, you can take heart, even if there seems to be lots of sheets, for, whatever happens, once the speaker get to the last sheet, the talk is over ..."
>
> James de Coquet

■ INTRODUCTION

The *introduction* is essential and vital to the success of the talk. This creates the atmosphere for the audience right from the start. Of course, one should not forget to thank the organizers for the opportunity to make a presentation at the meeting (this can advantageously be left to the end, as in a free paper session), but this is also the time when the speaker can show that he or she knows how to speak a little of the local language and is familiar with the history of the country or the town in which the meeting is taking place, that is, the speaker finds some way to establish a link between his talk and the audience. As in all introductions, there should be: 1) material to stimulate the curiosity of the audience, making them want to know more; and 2) pointers to indicate how the speaker is to achieve his or her goal and transmit the message. In practice, there is much to be gained from projecting a summary of the plan the speaker will take on the screen.

■ BODY OF THE TALK

Here, the speaker develops the thesis to be defended and then places it in relation to the antithesis. In support of the thesis, the speaker can use hard facts (evidence) with references, but what the audience really wants to know is how the speaker develops the ideas, especially the most original ideas. This is probably what distinguishes most a talk from a free paper presentation. Although the talk is structured, the structure is not as clearly defined, as the IMRAD structure does not apply here at all.

The number of ideas should be limited; two to three are enough. Too much information might distract and make the audience lose their train of thought. The speaker should select the main themes essential to the understanding of the topic, divide the talk into different sections, each corresponding to a different idea, and determine an appropriate and logical rhythm from one idea to the next, according to their importance and the time allotted to the talk.

Examples and comparisons should be extensively used to illustrate the ideas, but they must remain concrete: philosophical digressions and epilogues should be avoided. Clarity and conciseness are essential. Finding something that hits home with the audience in whatever domain, but in keep-ing with individual ideas, is always a strong point that goes down well and will contribute to the success of the presentation. References should be generously used to support the themes developed.

Transitions should be short. The end of each section should be clearly demarcated before going on to the next. A classic rhetorical technique is to lead the audience to something new by a comparison with something old that they are already familiar with.

■ CONCLUSION

This is the final act of the thesis/antithesis/synthesis. In contrast to the conclusion of the free paper presentation, the conclusion of a talk can (and should) make use of more general or universal concepts ("truths") with original or even philosophical extrapolations. In order to illustrate the message, contemporary problems can be alluded to, but care should be taken not to adopt a stance as regards political or social problems in the host country.

2
VISUAL AIDS

A lecture can be delivered with or without visual aids. Doing so without them is often dreaded by the person called upon to deliver a talk so that visual aids are used by and large. However, speaking without visual aids is an art form much sought after by the organizers and public. Without any visual aid, speakers must concentrate harder on what they say as all they have is words to get their message across.

If the speaker chooses to do the talk with visual aids, he or she can choose to use slides (or their computer equivalent), or overhead transparencies, which are often well suited to lectures.

■ SLIDES

As regards the slides, the same rules discussed above apply here: parsimonious use of text, and, here more than elsewhere, generous use of photographs, tables, graphs, etc. Using a double projection is a good idea if on one side the author shows data and on the other, a photograph. Another possibility is to put the summary on one side which remains there throughout the talk.

■ OVERHEAD TRANSPARENCIES

Although usually less elaborate than slides, overheads are another valuable visual aid. While they might appear to be less colorful and monotonous, they distract the audience less, but nonetheless require precise rules to be adhered to. One must be sure, however, that they will be seen in a large auditorium.

Design

Overheads are still too often poorly used and poorly designed. They often have the typical errors of poor slides. Overheads must be well spaced, without too many lines, columns, or text. Pollock has suggested no more than 12 lines and no more than 7 words per line. Both letters and figures must be sufficiently large in order to be seen from a distance: the size of the characters must be appropriate to the size of the room. The margins around the text of figures must be wide, in order to make the inside portion of the transparency easily legible.

Production

There are several ways of making overheads. As for slides, it is possible to photocopy texts, tables, or figures, for example, from textbooks. For texts, it is best to type them on an ordinary sheet of paper and then photocopy them on to the plastic overhead. If this is done, be sure to use heat-compatible overheads as the heat generated by photocopiers can melt the plastic sheet and ruin the machine. Overheads can also be produced by using the software used for slides such as Powerpoint™. In this case, the portrait layout should be used rather than landscape as, in our opinion (see below), this is more convenient. Finally, it is possible for the speaker to write directly on the overhead, at the same time as he or she speaks. In this case, only the essential, main words are written down for emphasis. They can then be circled or underlined to stress something or crossed out to highlight a negative effect.

Font and colors

When words are written by hand, attention must be paid to the thickness and color of the instrument used to write. When the color is pale, the letters show up poorly on the screen. This is because the light in the overhead projector is often intense and the background of the transparency is white. Black, dark blue, or dark red are recommended for the writing. Green and yellow should not be used. If a printer is used, once again the Helvetica or Arial fonts, size 18 or more, are preferred.

3
PRESENTATION

■ THE SPEAKER AND HIS OR HER ENVIRONMENT

The relationship between the speaker and the overhead projector is usually not very different from that which characterizes the use of slides. However, in reality, the situation can be very different. The best location for the overhead projector, for obvious optical reasons, is close to the screen, often on the stage itself. This, however, is not always possible, and sometimes the overhead projector is located elsewhere in the auditorium, usually in the first few rows of the audience. The speaker is then obliged either to leave the podium in order to stand next to the overhead projector, thus complicating the use of the microphone and changing the physical setup of the room and the audience, or to ask someone else to change the transparencies. As the maneuvers necessary to change each overhead are best performed by the speaker, this may create a problem. Whether it is the speaker, or someone else, special caution is required not to mix up the order of the sheets, or to drop them on the floor.

Even more often than the free paper session, a talk can be submitted to last-minute changes in schedule: absence of the speaker, delays in air travel, or tight or truncated schedules because of a political talk that has run over the allotted time. This means that the conference speaker has to think about what to do if this happens, and if the organizers ask him or her to make a change: this may mean *shortening or lengthening the talk by 5, 10, or even sometimes by 15 minutes.* Indeed, the duration of talks is much more flexible than that of the free paper sessions, where there are usually more than one speaker. Because these may be last-minute changes, the speaker must know the talk well and determine in advance which points or essential parts can or cannot be sacrificed without changing or distorting the message, whenever such a change is requested. Furthermore, sections that can be extended should also be land-marked, in advance and occasionally, a subsidiary or secondary topic can be added.

One good way of using the overhead sheets is to uncover each line or section sequentially, using an opaque piece of paper. As was described for slides, this can enliven the session somewhat (Fig. 13). This is why the portrait format is often preferable to the landscape format.

The orator can use a pen or any other pointed object, placed directly on the overhead sheet to highlight (emphasize) a word or phrase.

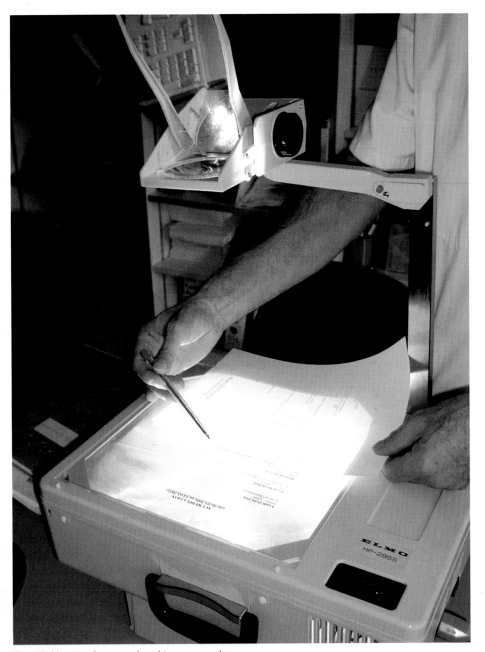

Fig. 13: How to show overhead transparencies.

Writing directly on the overhead sheet the elements that the orator wishes to stress is an interesting tactic for several reasons:

1. This adds an active component to the talk: the information is transmitted in real time.

2. This allows the orator to underline, in a different color, the word(s) or phrase(s) that seem to be the most important.

3. Information not originally on the sheet can be added, creating an element of suspense for those in the auditorium who are waiting for the solution to a problem or a difficult question.

4. Lastly, depending on the ability of the speaker, it is possible to draw directly on the screen, something which always attracts the attention of the audience.

To write directly on the overhead sheets, however, requires the use of special tools. The speaker should always check to make sure that they are available. A final word of caution is that the orator should be careful not to smudge the writing before it dries completely (which in fact may take several hours).

4
DISCUSSION

Normally, after a talk, neither comments nor questions are on the agenda. However, under specific conditions, particularly when the audience is small or selected, and if time allows, the moderator may ask for one or two comments or questions, or make his or her own.

THE PANEL DISCUSSION, ROUNDTABLE, SYMPOSIUM, AND COLLOQUIUM

The panel or roundtable discussion is a generic term that means that more than two persons (speaker and moderator) are on the stage at the same time. This may be part of a free paper session, or take place after several talks. It consists of inviting several people to give their opinion or comment on a specific topic (usually presented one after the other in the session preceding the roundtable session). The role of the moderator here is crucial, as he or she has to maintain order, make sure that each person at the roundtable on the podium gets to talk or comment, and at the same time ensure that a particular orator does not try to steal the show. Usually, at the end of the session, the moderator should summarize the information gleaned throughout the session. The moderator needs to federate during the debates and act as a "sage" when it comes to the synthesis or summary at the end of the session. Symposiums and colloquiums are simply other names for the roundtable format. As such, they should abide by the same rules.

1
CONCEPTION

Here the situation differs somewhat from other forms of communication because several speakers, together with the moderator, take the floor successively, usually, but not always, on a single theme. The speakers are called panelists. The choice of panelists is determined by their expertise on the topic(s) addressed. The relationship between the panelists, the moderator, and the audience differs somewhat from that of the free paper session or the talk. Because of this difference in the composition of the actors and setup, exchanges between the panelists and the audience are usually easier. The personalities of the different panelists may be a special, dynamic factor, specific to panel discussions. On the other hand, it is of the utmost importance to keep the talks and the sequence organized, which underscores the crucial role of the moderator in this form of communication. A disorganized or poorly conducted panel discussion will result in chaos and incomprehension of the topic, the opinions of the panelists, as well as the conclusions or recommendations.

Normally the organizers of the meeting or the moderator plan the topics with their specific titles and determine the order as well as the duration of the specific topics and talks of a well-organized panel discussion. Sometimes, however, only the title is indicated by the organizers. In this case, the moderator has a vital role which involves: 1) organizing the talks as well as the debate (with specific topics and time limits); and 2) contacting each of the panelists. If the moderator does not do so, then the panelists themselves have to get together beforehand to organize the session themselves. The goal, of course, is to harmonize the talks, yet avoid repetition or talking about topics that do not appear to be relevant to the others.

■ THE PREDOMINANT ROLE OF THE MODERATOR

Usually, each of the panelists is called to the podium in turn; none of the talks are followed directly by any discussion. Most of the time, the panelists are seated at a table on the other side of the stage. If not, at the end of the last presentation, the moderator asks all the panelists to sit at the same table. The moderator then asks several questions, or asks the audience to do so. A particular aspect of the panel discussion or roundtable (panelists seated around the table) is that each panelist is invited in turn to answer a specific question or to give their opinion concerning the same topic.

A second way of planning a panel discussion or roundtable is to have a debate on a given topic without any previous individual presentations: once everyone is seated, the moderator conducts the panel discussion or roundtable as above.

A third possibility is that the moderator is the person who presents: usually this is the way case reports or surgical vignettes are done. The moderator shows a case that poses some particular problems and then asks the panelists, one after another, what they think or would have done in this specific case. The audience then has a chance to intervene.

Independently of the type of panel (or roundtable), this mode of communication differs from the free paper session by the predominant weight given to the discussion, as opposed to the time devoted to individual contributions. Furthermore, it is the moderator, rather than someone in the audience, who usually leads the discussion. The discussion has no preset structure or time constraints (except that of the entire session). The moderator is free to choose the questions, the order in which the speakers respond, and whether and when the audience intervenes. Usually the discussion period is divided into several parts. First, the moderator summarizes the strong or essential points of the presentations, selecting (if only for sake of politeness) at least one point by speaker. This summary must be as brief as possible, but complete, highlighting the well-established facts, clearly setting out the controversies or where questions remain. Next, the moderator asks the questions. Usually the first question goes to the first panelist and then to each in turn, following a sequential order, at least for the first question. The following questions are asked starting with another speaker, but the order remains basically the same. The questions the moderator poses to the panelists usually concern the specific topic that the speaker addressed in his or her talk, then the same question (or a similar question) is asked to each member of the panel to see whether they agree or not. It is essential that the moderator knows the topic well and that the question(s) pinpoint the specific interesting details: if the questions are too general, the panelist will have a tendency to elaborate on minor elements and go off at a tangent. In order that all the tricky or interesting topics come to the floor, the replies of each panelist should be brief and to the point. The moderator can also ask the audience if they want to ask any questions or make any comments. In the same manner, each panelist will be asked by the moderator to give his or her opinion; once again, short answers are essential for a successful session. At the end of the session, the moderator draws the conclusions, after summarizing the remarks of each speaker.

The way questions are asked or comments are made does not differ from that discussed in the chapter on free papers.

THE POSTER

The poster is regarded with contempt by some sections of the medical profession, especially surgeons, who seem to think that a paper that was accepted as a poster is a failure.

The reasons why posters continue to get bad publicity include:
1. Making a poster is considered more difficult, constraining, and expensive than slides, even though the procedures for doing so have evolved greatly and have become much simpler.
2. Acceptance of a poster is considered to be compensation for an original presentation that was refused as a free paper.
3. Posters are often poorly exploited. If the author or the public are not present at the allotted or designated time for the discussion, no exchange of ideas is possible. Absence or poor motivation on the part of the author or the public may be related to organizational difficulties such as a conflict in the timing (parallel sessions) or the location of the posters, because they are either decentralized or set aside.
4. There is also the problem of cultural reticences because the time when the author is required to be present often coincides with the noon or lunch break. In some countries, especially in France, mealtimes are considered sacred! The breaks for lunch or coffee is also a key moment for people to meet and discuss other business.

In our opinion, the poster is an excellent means of communication, with undeniable advantages. In some meetings, posters are the main event as up to 85% of the presentations are accepted as posters, compared with only 15% as free papers! Once any communication has been accepted by a selection committee, the scientific value of a poster should be the same as a free paper. A poster presentation should have the same value and impact on a CV. The problem often stems from the fact that financial obligations (to make a congress a financial success, the organizers sometimes lower the standards of acceptance in order to guarantee a higher attendance) take precedence over quality. This tendency, however, has to be overcome and the surgical community should not only give posters the attention they deserve, but actually encourage them!

1
CONCEPTION

The way in which a poster is designed is important. A poster should attract the attention of any passerby. The authors should be beside the poster in order to be able to provide more details about it and answer any questions, whether they pertain to the contents or to the form.

There are at least two differences between the poster and the free paper:

1. The poster is simultaneously and directly in competition with the other posters, of which there may be many.

2. The audience is standing, not seated. This is why it is so important that the poster attracts the eye of the passerby. Moreover, posters should have a message which is obvious: it is understandable that the public wants a message that is clear, rapid, and attractive, so as not to become bored. With this in mind, a poster can be compared to a masterpiece in an art gallery: it should attract the public right from the start. As with the masterpiece in the gallery, the visitor usually wants to have more information. Therefore, details should not be given directly on the poster but orally. Details do have their place but should be in proportion to the rest of the information, while remaining accessible to the visitor. The visitor should not be distracted by useless details or complex data, which obscure the message and make it incomprehensible.

2
VISUAL SUPPORT

In parallel to the oral presentation, the poster may be divided into three parts: an *introduction*, a *body (methods and results)*, and a *conclusion*. A *discussion* section, that is a comparison between one's own results and those in the literature-with references-can be added, especially when one knows that there will be no formal oral presentation. The poster should have separate fields covering the allotted space, which, together, form a unit. This division is often directly related to the need to transport the poster with ease (see below). Each of the sections of the poster are composed of one or more fields.

Thus, there should be a title at the top, taking up the entire width of the poster (one line), followed by the names of the authors of the study (complete address with telephone, fax, and e-mail). The title, in a large point size, must be eye-catching, not only by its size and position, but also by its content, which has to capture the attention of passersby. When asked for by the organizers, the authors can put a summary under the title, usually on the left. The *introduction* clearly formulates the goals of the study. The *methods* and *results* section must be amply illustrated, making use of figures, photographs, and graphs, rather than tables. Text should be avoided. The poster must be visual. The *conclusion* (the *message*) should have a prominent position.

■ LAYOUT OF THE FIELDS

The fields of the poster can be arranged in several ways (Fig. 14). Because there is usually little room to stand back, and given that viewing is in a one-way direction to avoid too much milling about, the poster should be laid out in landscape format, with texts to be read vertically. This explains why the overall order of the fields should also be vertical. In order to facilitate reading, the fields should be arranged chronologically, from top to bottom.

The lowest fields of the poster, especially if the bottom of the poster is near the floor, are not easily seen, especially when there are many viewers. If there is a choice, the poster should be placed at least 40 cm above the floor.

In practice

Three examples of posters are given in Figure 14. The first two are landscape presentations, the most common. The conclusion can be put either at the bottom on the right, if a chronological order seems preferable (Fig. 14a), or in the middle of the poster, when the authors want the conclusion to stand out (Fig. 14b). The alternative is the "portrait" mode, which is much less frequently used (Fig. 14c).

Figure 15 shows a poster produced using Word.

a: Layout of the fields in a poster in the landscape format: 4 lines, 4 columns.

b: Poster layout in the landscape format with the conclusion in the middle.

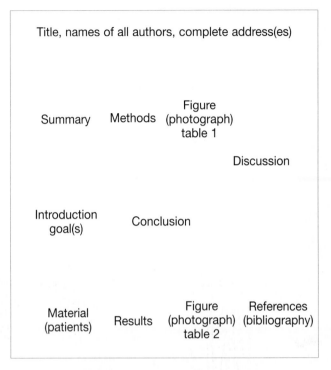

Title, names of all authors, complete address(es)

Summary   Methods   Figure
(photograph)
table 1

Discussion

Introduction
goal(s)   Conclusion

Material
(patients)   Results   Figure   References
(photograph) (bibliography)
table 2

c: Layout of the fields in a poster in the portrait format.

Fig. 14: Layout of fields in different forms of posters: a) landscape presentation; b) landscape presentation with conclusion in the middle of the poster; c) poster in the portrait mode.

3
PRESENTATION

At most congresses, some form of oral presentation is planned for the posters. Although how this is done differs somewhat from one congress to another, the author should remain near his or her poster for a given period of time. This mandatory presence ensures contact between the speaker and the public. This allows the visitor to discuss directly with the author(s) without any third party intervention, allowing at the same time an exchange of ideas and information under more intimate, and certainly more specific, conditions. Moreover, an advantage of the poster presentation is that there is no real time limit, or restriction on the number of questions or number of people who speak with the author. This system is certainly convivial. The range of questions can be very

CONVERSION FROM CYCLOSPORIN TO FK506 IN ADULT LIVER TRANSPLANTATION: RESULTS FROM A NORTH AMERICAN AND EUROPEAN SERIES

Nazia Malekkiani [1,2,3], Francois Durand [2], Jacques Bernuau [2], Michael A Heneghan [2], Janet E Tuttle-Newhall [1], Jacques Belghiti [2], and Pierre-Alain Clavien [1,3]
[1] Division of Transplantation and Hepatobiliary Surgery, Department of Surgery, Duke University Medical Center, Durham, NC/USA. [2] Department of Hepatology and Surgery Beaujon Hospital, Clichy, France and [3] Department of Visceral Surgery and Transplantation, University Hospital of Zurich, Switzerland

Abstract

Although Cyclosporin (CyA) remains an important drug in transplantation, side effects have limited its use. Conversion to FK506 is common practice in presence of toxicity of CyA. We evaluated the results of conversion from CyA to FK506 in a North American (Duke University) and a European (Clichy) liver transplant center. From January 1991 to September 1999, 620 liver transplantations has been performed in these centers.

Results: A total of 94 patients were converted from a CyA to a FK506 regimen following liver transplantation. The demographic characteristics and immunosuppressive regimens (including CyA, azathioprine and prednisone) were comparable in both centers. The main indication for conversion (in 47 (50%) of patients) was steroid-resistant acute cellular rejection (ACR). 92% of these patients had no recurrent rejection, while 8% developed chronic rejection (CR) despite conversion. 9 % (n=9) of patients on CyA had chronic rejection prior to conversion to FK506. Except for one case, each patient has responded to conversion with a current well functioning graft. The mean serum bilirubin level of these patients was 8.7mg/dl before conversion and 2.1mg/dl 6 months after conversion (P=0.021). A novel episode of rejection occurred in 4.5% patients during the follow up (mean= 30 months). Nine patients were converted for unsuccessful decrease in steroid dosage. 6 of these patients were steroid-free one year after conversion. 24 % (n=23) of patients were converted for nephrotoxicity. The serum creatinine value in these patients decreased from 167+ 36 mmol/l to 119+ 28 one year after conversion (P<.006). 11% (n=11) were converted for neurotoxicity. Significant improvement was observed in all patients with headache or tremor (p=0.01). Conversion to FK506 has no effect on seizures or memory loss. 2 patients were converted for hyperlipidemia. Serum cholesterol and triglyceride normalized in both cases within 6 months. Conversion had no effect on arterial hypertension and diabetes.

Conclusion: Conversion to FK506 is beneficial for a number of indications related to CyA-related toxicity except for seizures, memory loss, arterial hypertension and diabetes. Novel strategies should be developed in these situations.

Background

Cyclosporine (CyA) is often use as maintaining immunosuppressive regimen

In some cases (CyA) is associated with:
- poorly tolerated sides effects
- development of steroid-resistant acute or chronic rejection

Alternative immunosupression should be sometimes considered.

Aim

To evaluate the results of conversion from CsA to FK506 in 2 separate centers in the US and Europe

Patients & Methods

- From January 1990 to September 1999

- 94 allografts were converted in a North American (Duke University) and European Center (Hopital Beaujon)

- Primary immunosuppression regimens and rejection treatment were comparable in both centers

- Indications for conversion;
  → CsA induced side effects
  → Steroids resistant acute rejection
  → Chronic ductopenic rejection

Results

Survival

- 2 years Survival	Duke	Clichy
• Graft	88%	96%
• Patient	92%	96%

Conversion for steroid-resistant acute or chronic rejection

Indication for Conversion	Total	Resolved	Improvement	No effect
	Number of patients and percentage of total (%)			
Acute cellular rejection	47 (50)	43 (91.5)	0	4 (8.5)
Chronic rejection	9 (9)	6 (66)	2 (22)	1 (11)

Conversion for side effects

Indication for Conversion	Total	Resolved	Improvement	No effect
	Number of patients and percentage of total (%)			
Nephrotoxicity	23 (24)	9 (39)	6 (26)	8 (34)
Neurotoxicity	11 (11)	7 (63)	1 (9)	3 (27)
Failure to decrease steroid dosage	9 (9)	6 (66)	0	3 (33)
Elevated LFTs of unknown etiology	6 (6)	2 (33)	1 (16)	3 (50)
Gingival hypertrophy	1	1	0	0
Hyperlipidemia	2	2	0	0
Diabetes	3	0	0	3
Hypertension	16 (17)	0	0	16 (100)

Conclusions

Conversion from CsA to FK506 is an appropriate paradigm for:

→ Graft rescue in case of acute resistant or chronic rejection
→ Treatment of a variety of side effects post transplant

large and, in particular, they can deal with details that might have been left aside in a free paper presentation for the sake of time.

According to the organization of the congress, there are several ways to comment on or present a poster:

1. At some meetings, the poster is put up and stays posted for a specific period of time only, not the entire duration of the meeting. In addition, a specific time period is allotted to the author (or presenter) to stay beside the poster, in order to answer questions posed by the people viewing the poster.

2. At other meetings, a jury, designated by the organizers, passes from one poster to another at a time scheduled in advance. In this setting, the author is either free to answer any specific questions asked by a member of the jury, or is asked to comment on the poster in front of the jury: in the latter case, it is recommended to comment on the poster field by field. The points of the discussion can be introduced by highlighting a particular topic which the author feels warrants further discussion. During the presentation, the author should look alternately not only at the president, but also at the other members of the jury. Speak softly-the people are very close to you-and slowly. Be prepared to be interrupted at any time by the listeners. Questions should be answered very briefly but precisely, and the orator should then continue the presentation, making sure not to lose track of where he or she left off when the question was asked. In contrast to the free paper session, minutes do not count, but the discussion should not be prolonged or the subject deviated from. Preparing oneself for questions about the contents as well as on the form of the poster is a wise precaution.

3. A third formula, used more and more worldwide, is for the organizers to designate a discussant or someone who, after studying a group of posters, summarizes them in public. The discussant is the person who gives the talk before the audience, who can then ask the authors questions or make comments. The discussant, however, no longer intervenes.

4. Most often, the author will be asked to present the poster to the audience in an abbreviated form. In this setting, the comments (on the poster) are very brief, probably the shortest duration of any form of oral communication (usually 3 minutes at the most). This limited time explains why this form of communication is quite difficult.

The short presentation resembles that of the free paper presentation in terms of the *situation* in which the orator finds himself or herself (room with a moderator and audience), usually with the possibility of showing one, two, or exceptionally three slides. However, there are several constraints that distinguish between the two. The short duration of the presentation does not allow the speaker to keep to the complete IMRAD structure. The orator, after a short introduction (one or two sentences), should limit his presentation to the main thrust of the message. The title, for instance, is already on the poster, in the program, and will probably be announced by the moderator. There is therefore no need either to state it, or put it on the slides.

The number of slides should never exceed the number of minutes (3 minutes should ideally correspond to two slides, three at the most). The goal here is not to try to cram a 10-minute presentation into three slides. Only one or two slides can be used for the methods and/or the results. This means that if two are used for the methods there is only one for the results, and vice versa.

Here, more than elsewhere, it is essential that the conclusion or the practical consequences are announced in front of the audience in a room with the lights on. The comments can be addressed by the speaker in the discussion period which should also last close to 3 minutes: there is no need to put them on a slide. As time is limited, and if the speaker absolutely wants to communicate complementary information, this can be done by making handouts available to the audience (including data not shown on the poster, figures, graphs, and tables as well as references).

Questions most often asked and practical recommendations for posters:
1. What are the size and orientation of the posters?
Usually the sizes of the posters are limited and dictated by the organizers. The poster can be in landscape or portrait. The dimensions most often used are:
180 cm x 120 cm in Europe.
12 x 24 inches in the USA.

2. When should the poster be set up?
Very often, the organizers lay down very strict rules for putting up and taking down the posters, usually because one batch of posters has to be changed from one day to the next, sometimes from one session to the next during the same day. Putting up a poster can actually take some time and this has to be planned in advance. The removal of the poster usually takes place according to a very specific time frame, otherwise the poster may be taken down, destroyed, and/or lost.

Whatever the type of presentation of the poster, the organizers can reward the best posters in two ways: by either awarding a prize and/or putting them into a special plenary session, a selected poster session which should fit into the schedule in a prime spot, sometimes called the "president's session."

Notwithstanding, posters do have a certain number of shortcomings or pitfalls.

Transportation

Putting or pasting all the information on one single sheet of paper or cardboard according to the final required or recommended dimensions sometimes creates transportation problems, because the final dimensions of the rolled up document take up considerable space (at least 120 cm [see insertion frame]). The alternative solution is to divide the poster up into several smaller units that are more easily transportable, but then the poster has to be mounted in the space allocated and before the presentation. Special attention must be paid in order that the final mounted poster remains professional and is not squint. This technique calls for a bit of experience and emphasizes the need to calculate the size of each unit in order to ensure the final harmony.

Sometimes the authors have the unpleasant surprise of discovering that the dimensions of the poster boards do not correspond to those specified in the instructions to the authors. In that case one has to adapt to the situation. While most often the material needed can be found at the venue for the meeting, sometimes it may be necessary to find scissors, glue, tape, or tacks, etc.

OTHER FORMS OF COMMUNICATION

1
VIDEO WITH COMMENTS

A video with commentary is an excellent means of communication. It seems easy to do. This is probably why this apparently simple means of communication is often poorly used. Animation is well suited describing the way to examen a patient, an operative or endoscopic technique, etc.

The video may or may not have a sound track. The main advantage of a sound track is optimal synchronization between sound and pictures. There is no hesitation or repetition, and it is easy to transmit a message in a foreign language. The disadvantage is that if the author does not do the commentary in real time, the presentation is not "live", and one may then even ask why the speaker has come to stand in front of the audience if he or she does not speak! More annoying is the fact that the speaker often wants to make comments and, if he or she does not know where the silent sequences are, this can rapidly lead to comments being made over the commentary.

In contrast, a silent film, without a sound track, is an advantage in that it makes the video presentation seem more of a live event, and the speaker does what a speaker is there to do. The main difference, compared with an unanimated visual aid like slides, is that a video is made up of images that run at a constant speed, and this not allow for long comments. If the comments take too much time, the sequence for which they were intended may well have passed and therefore confusion may set in. This is one of the reasons why, contrary to what one might imagine, the comments that accompany a video have to be prepared and rehearsed in advance, just as if this was another type of presentation, and the speaker was to give a talk about a similar topic.

The following are useful recommendations:

1. For the same reasons as those given for the other visual aids such as

slides, the introduction and conclusion are best delivered orally, with the room lights on, without any visual aid.

2. The rules that apply to the use of the pointer are the same as for any other circumstances.

3. If the actual length of the film is longer than what the organizers had planned for or allowed (although this should be avoided), one has the possibility of fast-forwarding some of the sequences concentrating on one or several points of interest.

4. Last, video clips may be inserted into presentations produced with a computer. The combination of slides and video is an excellent method of presentation, but should be perfectly rehearsed and planned in advance.

2
THE INVITED COMMENT

A particular form of oral presentation is what might be called a planned commentary, in which the speaker has the role of critic or debater, also called a discussant. The material must be well prepared in advance. For this preparation, the topic must either be well known already or studied. The scientific committee has the important task of communicating the summary or better still, the entire manuscript, well in advance so that the discussant has the necessary time to prepare his or her intervention.

The discussants should construct the critique in the following manner:

1. Thank the organizers for giving him or her the opportunity to make a critique.

2. Congratulate the speaker and then underline the strong, original, points of the presentation.

3. Send a reminder to the audience concerning the methods used and the results of the work, emphasizing the positive points.

4. List the comments and/or questions, in order to indicate to the speaker whether to take notes.

5. Highlight the points upon which the discussant is in agreement, using the literature or personal experience in support of his or her viewpoint.

6. Argue the salient points with which the discussant is not in agreement.

This is the prompt to start off the discussion.

Whenever necessary, the discussant can use some form of visual aid, generally speaking, one slide. However, the discussant must not lose sight of his or her role, and not take the place of the speaker. The function of the discussant is to emphasize and highlight the qualities of the communication and stimulate the beginning of the discussion.

3
BLACKBOARD
OR PAPER BOARD
(WHITE BOARD, FLIP CHART)

Blackboard, white boards, or flip charts are methods of presentation well suited to small gatherings, in small rooms, essentially because the boards cannot be seen from far away.

■ BLACKBOARD

Presenting a report in this manner is a lively experience because it allows the speaker to animate the talk. In actual fact, the speaker has the possibility of creating his visual aid right in front of the audience. Watching someone actually drawing or writing down the essential messages on a board is an enlivening experience and adds greatly to the delivery of the message. Several types of presentations are well suited to this. This is especially the case for anatomy lessons, or talks about specific anatomical details as related to surgical techniques, physiology diagrams, to name just a few. This implies, however, that the speaker is an excellent artist, and that the preparations and necessary rehearsals have been done well in advance.

■ FLIP CHART

The flip chart can be used like a white board, with the difference that it is not necessary to erase what is on the board, or may be used in the same way as overheads. All the speaker has to do, therefore, is to flip over the sheets one after the other, and then color, underline, or highlight in some other manner the important or essential points. These data can also be added while the speaker is talking, on a background sheet prepared in advance. Another advantage of this type of presentation is that the speaker can go back one or more sheets whenever, and as much as, he or she so desires.

4
LITERATURE REVIEWS

The role of literature review sessions is to look at and analyze the most important papers published since the last session. This form of presentation is very dependent on the relevance of the comments made on the paper. One of the most frequent faults with this type of presentation is that the speaker places too much emphasis on the technical aspects of the paper, giving too many details on the material and methods, and goes through all the results in detail, essentially repeating what may be gleaned from actually reading the entire article. Not enough is said about whether the information contained in the article is pertinent or not, with respect to its place in the framework of the overall theme, its place and impact with respect to the rest of the literature, and the current state of the art. In order to do this, the presenter must have extensive knowledge and be well read in the field under discussion.

■ THE PRESENTATION

It is not usually necessary to give the full bibliographical reference, just the topic and the journal is enough. The complete reference, however, should be available on the visual aid that is used (overhead, slide, or handout). The reasons for doing the study, usually found in the introduction of the paper, should be announced clearly and concisely. The material and methods section can usually be summarized by one or two tables, on which the presenter comments. The same holds true for the principal results. The conclusion of the authors should be given as simply as possible. Most important is what follows, the original part of this type of presentation: critical comments on the paper, as much on the form, style, comprehensibility, and quality, as on the contents. This criticism opens the door for the discussion.

■ ANALYSIS

For original research papers, the analysis should follow the points defined by M. Evans and A. Pollock (*Br J Surg.* 1985;72:256-260):

1. *Design and conducting of trials:* Definition of the sample, specific inclusion and exclusion criteria, report of risk factors, complete description of therapeutic regimens, obtaining informed consent, definition of outcome measures and end points, calculation of the number of patients necessary, patient consent, description of randomization method, blinding in order to evaluate results, consecutive patients, and recording of side effects.

2. *Analysis of results:* Analysis of all patients entered in the trial (the number of exclusions should not exceed 10% of the total number of included patients) and outcome of those patients who were not randomized or withdrawn secondarily, presence of a table showing the comparability of the groups studied, stratification of risk factors, statistical analysis, and use of appropriate statistical tests.

3. *Presentation of the text:* Accurate title, correspondence between summary and the body of the article, reproducibility of methods, commented presentation of all data, credibility of results, do the results justify the conclusions? Are the references correct in number and in quality (year, volume, and pages)? Lastly, are the results clinically applicable, especially as regards the use of confidence intervals?

WHAT TO DO WHEN SOMETHING GOES WRONG OR NOT AS PLANNED

1
VISUAL AID

– The visual aid you had planned to use is not available or is not working properly. This is the case when the slide projector (or video) stops running, there is no slide projector (or video), or the slides have not been delivered to the room in time.

Two solutions are possible:

1) Use another type of material made available by the organizers (for instance, overheads, white board or flip chart); or

2) Speak without any visual aid. Both solutions, especially the latter, require that the structure and contents of the talk that be well known to the speaker and that he or she has taken the precaution of taking along a hard paper copy of the talk.

– The slides are upside down, sideways or inverted left to right, one or more slides may be missing, or not in the order you had planned. Last, the slides are not yours.

There is often more than one way of finding a solution. If the slides are upside down, on their side, or inverted left to right, the speaker has to keep calm, and just ask for the slides to be put into the correct position. In the other situations, it may be a bit more difficult to solve the problem, especially if you are not familiar with slide projectors. Here, it is best not to insist on getting the slides into the correct order, just go on with the talk (usually the audience does not know the order or the number of slides you had planned on anyway). These potential mishaps underline the need to try to project your slides (or run your video) entirely before the beginning of the session, if possible with the same equipment and in the room where the talk will be given. Increasingly often, the organization will integrate your slide show into a network and it will be transmitted directly to the auditorium or room in which your talk is being delivered. This is the ideal situation. Otherwise, you may be required to use you own portable, but this may take some time to hook up. It is therefore advisable to get your computer running just before the time slot scheduled for your talk. Another delay may be caused when it is necessary to reboot your computer once it has been hooked up. In this case, it is more important than ever to prepare and deliver your introduction with the lights on and without any visual aid (while the computer is rebooting). Tell the room staff not to show the screen during this set up as everyone will look at the screen (especially if it is in a foreign language) and not listen to what you have to say.

2
LIGHTING

– The lights remain on during your talk. Do not shout at the staff or the organizers, just keep on talking as if nothing was wrong, with the lights on, and politely ask that the lights be switched off.

– Or, in contrast, the room is completely dark, you cannot find the podium, or the pointer, or see the notes you had planned to read. This, once again, underscores the need to know the text and the contents of your talk sufficiently well to get by without lights. Rest assured that the staff will do their best to accommodate, and they or someone in the audience might even find a little handheld light to bail you out.

3
MICROPHONE

– The microphone does not work:

1. If the size of the room allows, it usually is enough to raise one's voice and speak louder. If the room is not full, the moderator (or the speaker) can ask the audience to move forward into the front rows.

2. If the room is too big, the moderator must do his or her job and get the organizers to find a solution as soon as possible. In the meantime, do not wait in silence or argue with the staff, but remain calm and do as best you can under these circumstances.

– The microphone crackles or deforms the speaker's voice:

1. The speaker should check the position of the microphone in relation to his or her mouth, and find the right distance so that the problem disappears.

2. The speaker should check that there is no metal or other objects nearby which might interfere with the microphone or radio transmission. This is especially true of metal objects that the speaker may have in his or her pockets.

3. If the problem persists, the speaker must be prepared to speak without the microphone (as if it were not working at all).

4
POINTER

Either the speaker cannot get it to work (it should have been tested beforehand), or help can be asked from the staff or the moderator.

In any case, the speaker should refrain from complaining about the poor organization or lack of it. Everyone in the room will share the same frustration and it is no good adding to the confusion. Just keep on talking as if nothing were wrong, do not frown or scorn, smile and, if possible, try to find some way to make a joke of it. Everything is on your side; it will go against you (as far as your image is concerned) to appear as a poor player. You must keep the situation under control.

All these problems stress the importance of coming to the room in advance, to try everything out to make sure that all is working properly beforehand, and ask for ample information on how to use the instruments, lighting, slide projection, etc.

THE SPEAKER'S APPEARANCE

In order to adhere to correct protocol, the speaker should pay close attention to his or her appearance: he or she should be well groomed and dressed appropriately.

The speaker should always inquire as to whether special dress is required. If in any doubt, remain traditional, a dark gray or black suit with a fairly neutral colored tie for men and an executive suit for women should be the basic dress.

Remember to take a handkerchief with you to wipe your forehead in case of excessive heat, your nose in case you have a cold, and mouth and nose in case you sneeze.

If, in spite of all our recommendations, you still want to read your notes or your text if you are in a foreign country, for example, do not forget your glasses.

When you begin to speak, whether you are a speaker, the moderator or from the floor (to ask a question or make a comment for instance), breathe slowly and keep your head high; do not slouch, in particular, do not lean on the lectern, stay in the same place and do not move back and forth, play with your hands, shuffle your feet, or fidget with the microphone or the pointer.

Adjust your voice according to the power of the microphone and the size of the room. Beware of speaking too close to the microphone as it will alter your voice, and the buzzing or shrill sound will annoy everyone to the point that they will have trouble listening to the talk and the message will be lost. By speaking too far away from the microphone, the speaker will not be heard.

Remember that no matter what else is happening, a smile will allow you to get out of most difficulties.

TIPS FOR YOUR TRIP

Never put your slides in your checked baggage: always carry them with you. Lost baggage (or even theft) would leave you in a very difficult spot. Think of carrying a paper copy of your text, slides, or notes. If you are making a computer presentation, it is a good idea to bring slides along just in case, especially when traveling to countries where up-to-date equipment may be lacking or fail.

As soon as you arrive, take a close look at the final version of the program to find out if there are any last-minute changes in the time schedule, the speakers, or the order of the presentations of the session. Any of these may be very different from what was planned originally.

1
JET LAG

Tiredness or, on the contrary, insomnia, gastrointestinal discomfort, and the inability to concentrate are all part of what is commonly called jet lag. These disorders are due to the difference between the time of your internal clock, and the external clock or the time of the country that you are traveling to.

In order to fight off this problem, let us review the data concerning the circadian rhythm in humans. The physiological cycle of what we might call the internal clock depends on external stimuli such as morning and evening light and noises (birds), the light cycle (day and night), meals (and drinks), everyday tasks and social events, and by finding out exactly what time of the day or night it really is (by taking a look at your watch for instance). Chronobiologists have taught us that when someone is cut off from all external stimuli, the internal clock no longer works on a 24-hour cycle, but rather a 25-hour cycle. Extending this to 26 to 28 hours is much easier than shortening it. In other words, it is easier to advance your internal clock than delaying it. This explains why it may be easier to adapt to traveling from east to west than from west to east. The rule of thumb is that it takes as many days to recuperate as the number of time zones you have traveled through.

Traveling from east to west

Flying from the east to the west coast of the United States, the time difference is never more than 4 hours. Flights can be had at any time of the day and this is usually not much of a problem. Traveling across the Pacific to Asia, or travelling to the USA from Europe, however, is a different story.

One way of trying to adjust your internal clock is to shift the time at which you go to sleep two to three days before you leave. If you usually go to sleep at 10 PM for instance, try staying up 1 hour more (until 11 PM), then until midnight and then until 1 AM. When you get to your destination, you have already adjusted to the equivalent of three time zones. This is especially true for people who need regular and fixed sleeping patterns. If not, it is important to avoid the temptation to go to bed as soon as you arrive in your hotel, just to catch up on what you may feel is lost sleep. This will just prolong the problem. Traveling from east to west, however, with a bit of persistence, can be easily overcome especially when there is still light outside, and if the city you are in has adequate evening and nightlife. Getting to bed later and later is fairly easy and with a bit of habit, you can get adjusted fairly easily.

Traveling from west to east

Most trips in this direction are overnight flights. Shifting the time you get up by one hour earlier every day for the two or three days before you leave is one way of trying to shift your internal clock. If the time away from home is less than the number of time zones you are traveling through, this may be enough. Taking a night ("red-eye") flight from the west to east coast of the United States is probably worse than traveling to Europe. The night you experience is just too short. When the flight lasts at least six or seven hours, however, another solution is to take a rapid-acting sleeping pill with a short half-life such as zolpidem as soon as you board the plane. Ask the hostess not to wake you up, even for the evening meal, but only for breakfast, put blinders on, insert ear plugs and ensure your head stays in a good position, usually with a cushion or inflatable pillow, and try to get as much sleep as the trip will allow.

In other words, you must try to adapt to the rhythm and habits of the country you travel to (mealtimes, social contacts, afternoon naps, etc). For short trips (lasting fewer days than the number of time zones you cross), it may be just as effective to stay within your own internal clock frame, going to sleep, and getting up, early or late, as necessary.

FURTHER READING

Barbier JH, Coiteux LP. La double projection simultanée des diapositives ou "le complexe de l'écureuil." *Presse Méd.* 1992;21:189-190.

Czeisler CA, Kronauer RK, Allan JS, Duffy JF, Jewett ME, Brown EN, Ronda JM. Bright light induction of strong (type 0) resetting of the human circadian pacemaker. *Science.* 1989;244:1328-1332.

Czeisler CA, Allan JS, Strogtz SH, Ronda JM, Sanches R, Rios CD, Freitag WF, Richardson GS, Kronauer RK. Bright light resets the human circadian pacemaker independent of the timing of the sleep-wake cycle. *Science.* 1986;233: 667-671.

Czeisler CA, Johnson MP, Duffy JF, Brown EN, Ronda JM, Kronauer RK. Exposure to bright light and darkness to treat physiologic maladaptation to night work. *N Engl J Med.* 1990;322:1253-1259.

Evans M, Pollock M. A score system for evaluating random control clinical trials of prophylaxis of abdominal surgical wound infection. *Br J Surg.* 1985;72: 256-260.

Fingerhut A. In: *Principles and Practice of Research. Strategies for Surgical Investigators.* 2nd edition. Edited by H Troidl, WO Spitzer, B McPeek, MDS Mulder, MF McKneally, AS Wedhsler, CM Balch. New York, NY: Springer-Verlag; 1991.

Hawkins C. *Speaking at Meetings in Research. How to Plan, Speak and write about it.* Berlin, Germany: Springer-Verlag; 1985 pp 60-84.

Hoff R. *I Can See You Naked.* New revised edition. Kansas City, Miss: Universal Press Syndicate Company; 1992.

McPeek B, Herfarth C. The longer talk. In: *Principles and Practice of Research. Strategies for Surgical Investigators.* 2nd edition. Edited by H Troidl, WO Spitzer, B McPeek, MDS Mulder, MF McKneally, AS Wedhsler, CM Balch. New York, NY: Springer-Verlag; 1991.

Mosteller F. Classroom and platform performance. *Am Stat.* 1980;34:11-17.

Pollock A, Evans M. In: *Principles and Practice of Research. Strategies for Surgical Investigators.* 2nd edition. Edited by H Troidl, WO Spitzer, B McPeek, MDS Mulder, MF McKneally, AS Wedhsler, CM Balch. New York, NY: Springer-Verlag; 1991.

Achevé d'imprimer sur les presses de l'Imprimerie BARNÉOUD
B.P. 44 - 53960 BONCHAMP-LÈS-LAVAL
Dépôt légal : février 2002 – N° d'imprimeur : 13042